# COMPLETE GUIDE TO CROHN'S DISEASE

A Comprehensive Handbook To Expert Strategies For Diagnosis, Treatment, Nutrition, Surgery, Lifestyle Management And Coping Techniques

**DEHART HAIRSTON**

© [DEHART HAIRSTON], [2024]

All rights reserved. No part of this publication may be reproduced, distributed, or transmitted in any form or by any means, including photocopying, recording, or other electronic or mechanical methods, without the prior written permission of the publisher, except in the case of brief quotations embodied in critical reviews and certain other noncommercial uses permitted by copyright law.

**DISCLAIMER**

This book's content is only intended for general informative purposes. At the time of writing, the author has taken every precaution to guarantee that the material is correct and current. Nevertheless, the author disclaims all explicit and implicit representations and guarantees about the availability, appropriateness, correctness, completeness, and usefulness of the material on these pages.

Since the author is not a licensed medical practitioner, the material in this book shouldn't be interpreted as medical advice. Before making any modifications to their diet, exercise regimen, or medical treatment, readers are urged to speak with a licensed healthcare provider.

Moreover, the author has no connection to any of the businesses, organizations, or people that are discussed in this book. Any mentions of goods, services, businesses, or people are purely informative and do not indicate endorsement or suggestion.

This book's content is entirely dependent on the author's expertise, study, and comprehension of the topic. Despite having taken reasonable care to offer correct information, the author disclaims all liability for any mistakes or omissions in the material as well as for any losses, harm, or damages resulting from using the information.

It is recommended that readers use their own judgment and discretion when applying the knowledge in this book to their own situations. The use or implementation of any material in this book may result in unfavorable repercussions, directly or indirectly, for which the author assumes no liability.

By reading this book, you agree to release and hold the author harmless from any claims, losses, liabilities, costs, or expenditures resulting from or related to the use of the information you get from it.

## Table of Contents

**CHAPTER 1** .................................................. 13
  Understanding Crohn's Disease .............................. 13
  What Is Crohn's Disease? .................................. 13
  Causes And Risk Factors ................................... 14
  Symptoms And Signs ........................................ 15

**CHAPTER 2** .................................................. 17
  Diagnosing Crohn's Disease ................................ 17
  Medical History And Physical Examination .................. 17
  Diagnostic Tests: Blood Tests, Imaging, Endoscopy ......... 18
    Blood tests ........................................... 18
    Imaging studies ....................................... 19
    Endoscopy ............................................. 21

**CHAPTER 3** .................................................. 23
  Treatment Options ......................................... 23
  Medications: Anti-Inflammatory, Immune Suppressors, Biologics .................................... 23
    Medications ........................................... 23
    Immune Suppressors: ................................... 24
  Lifestyle Changes: Diet, Exercise, Stress Management ................................................ 25

- Lifestyle Changes ................................................ 25
- Diet: ....................................................................... 25
- Exercise: ............................................................... 26
- Stress Management: ............................................ 26
- Surgery: When And Why ........................................ 27
  - Surgery ................................................................. 27
  - Forms of Surgery: ............................................... 28
  - Risks and Considerations: ................................. 28
- **CHAPTER 4** ............................................................ 31
  - Managing Symptoms .......................................... 31
  - Dealing With Flare-Ups ...................................... 31
  - Coping With Pain And Discomfort .................... 32
  - Nutritional Support ............................................. 34
- **CHAPTER 5** ............................................................ 37
  - Diet And Nutrition .............................................. 37
  - Foods To Avoid ................................................... 37
  - Foods To Include ................................................ 39
  - Meal Planning Tips ............................................. 42
    - 1. Maintain a Food Diary: ................................. 42
    - 2. Focus on Variety: ........................................... 42
    - 4. Consider Texture: .......................................... 43

    5. Remind Hydrated: ................................................43

    6. Plan for Snacks: ...................................................44

    7. Listen to Your Body: ............................................44

    8. Consult a Dietitian: ..............................................44

## CHAPTER 6 ................................................................45

    Living With Crohn's Disease ....................................45

    Maintaining Quality Of Life ....................................45

    Support Networks And Resources ..........................47

    Mental Health And Well-Being ................................48

## CHAPTER 7 ................................................................51

    Complications Of Crohn's Disease ..........................51

    Fistulas, Abscesses, And Strictures ........................51

    Malnutrition And Vitamin Deficiencies ...................53

    Osteoporosis And Bone Health ...............................55

## CHAPTER 8 ................................................................59

    Pregnancy And Crohn's Disease .............................59

    Fertility Issues ..........................................................59

    Pregnancy Management .........................................60

    Risks And Precautions ............................................61

## CHAPTER 9 ................................................................63

    Children And Crohn's Disease ................................63

    Pediatric Considerations ............................................. 63
    Growth And Development............................................ 64
    Treatment Approaches ................................................ 65
**CHAPTER 10** ....................................................................... 69
    Research And Future Perspectives............................. 69
    Advances In Crohn's Disease Research ................... 69
    Promising Therapies On The Horizon ..................... 71
    Advocacy And Awareness Efforts ............................ 73
    **CONCLUSION**.......................................................... 76
    **THE END** ................................................................... 79

## ABOUT THIS BOOK

This book "Crohn's Disease" is an invaluable resource for anybody living with this chronic ailment, providing a thorough explanation as well as practical advice for dealing with its difficulties. Chapter 1 introduces readers to the principles of Crohn's disease, including its etiology, symptoms, and risk factors. This fundamental understanding is required for people to detect and successfully treat the illness.

Chapter 2 digs into the diagnosis procedure, offering information on the numerous medical exams and testing needed to confirm Crohn's disease. Understanding these diagnostic processes enables people to seek immediate medical assistance and begin suitable treatment strategies.

One of this book's strongest points is Chapter 3, which delves into the many therapy choices for

Crohn's disease. Readers obtain vital ideas about comprehensively treating their disease, including drugs, lifestyle changes, and surgical procedures.

Chapter 4 discusses the daily problems of living with Crohn's Disease, including practical suggestions for managing symptoms and preserving nutritional balance. This section is especially useful for those who are experiencing flare-ups and looking for solutions to relieve suffering.

As discussed in Chapter 5, diet and nutrition play an important part in Crohn's disease management. Readers may maximize their dietary choices to meet their health objectives by following thorough instructions on which foods to include and which to avoid, as well as meal planning suggestions.

Chapter 6 dives into the psychological elements of living with Crohn's disease, highlighting the significance of preserving quality of life, connecting with support networks, and putting mental health first.

Furthermore, in Chapter 7, this book discusses probable Crohn's Disease consequences, providing readers with the information they need to detect and successfully manage these issues. Chapters 8 and 9 include particular information on pregnancy and pediatric issues, responding to the specific requirements of people at various stages of life.

Finally, Chapter 10 delves into continuing research and future views on Crohn's Disease, emphasizing breakthroughs in treatment choices and advocacy initiatives. This section instills hope and empowers readers by providing information on developing medicines and activities targeted at improving outcomes for Crohn's patients.

In short, "Crohn's Disease" is more than simply a book; it's a lifeline for anyone trying to understand the complexity of this ailment. Its thorough coverage, practical ideas, and empowering attitude make it an invaluable resource for patients, caregivers, and healthcare professionals alike.

# CHAPTER 1

## Understanding Crohn's Disease

### What Is Crohn's Disease?

Crohn's disease is a chronic inflammatory ailment that mostly affects the digestive system, although it may affect any organ of the body. It is classed as inflammatory bowel disease (IBD), alongside ulcerative colitis. Unlike ulcerative colitis, which affects just the colon and rectum, Crohn's disease may affect any part of the gastrointestinal (GI) tract, including the mouth and anus.

The actual etiology of Crohn's disease is unclear, however, it is thought to be a mix of genetic, environmental, and immunological factors. The immune system, which typically defends the body against infection, erroneously assaults healthy tissue in the digestive tract, causing inflammation and damage. This persistent inflammation may cause a variety of symptoms and consequences over time.

## Causes And Risk Factors

While the exact etiology of Crohn's disease is unknown, various variables are believed to contribute to its development. Genetics plays an important role since those who have a family history of the condition are more likely to get it themselves. Certain genetic variations may make certain people more likely to develop Crohn's disease when exposed to particular environmental factors.

Environmental variables can influence the development of Crohn's disease. Diet, smoking, and exposure to certain illnesses or toxins may all raise the likelihood of getting the disorder. However, not everyone exposed to these conditions develops Crohn's disease, suggesting that additional factors, including as genetic predisposition, play an important role.

## Symptoms And Signs

Crohn's disease may produce a broad variety of symptoms that vary in intensity and may appear and go over time. Common symptoms include stomach discomfort, diarrhea, rectal bleeding, weight loss, exhaustion, and fever. These symptoms may have a substantial influence on someone's quality of life, causing physical pain and mental suffering.

In addition to digestive symptoms, Crohn's disease may cause consequences such as arthritis, skin rashes, eye irritation, and liver dysfunction. The particular symptoms experienced might vary depending on where and how severe the inflammation is in the digestive system.

Early identification and treatment of Crohn's disease are critical for controlling symptoms and avoiding complications. If you have prolonged stomach discomfort, diarrhea, or other troubling symptoms, you should visit a healthcare expert for an accurate diagnosis and treatment plan. Crohn's disease is a chronic disorder, but with careful treatment, many people may live productive lives with little interruptions from their symptoms.

# CHAPTER 2

## Diagnosing Crohn's Disease

## Medical History And Physical Examination

When it comes to diagnosing Crohn's Disease, the process often begins with a complete medical history review and physical examination. This stage is critical because it helps healthcare specialists to better understand your symptoms, any previous medical illnesses, family history, and lifestyle variables that may be influencing your present health.

During the medical history review, your healthcare practitioner will inquire about your symptoms, including stomach discomfort, diarrhea, weight loss, and weariness. They will also question your medical history, such as any past gastrointestinal difficulties, surgeries, or drugs you are currently taking.

It is critical that you offer honest and complete answers to these questions so that your healthcare professional can make an accurate diagnosis.

Following the medical history review, a thorough physical examination is performed. This exam may involve palpating your abdomen for discomfort or swelling, listening to your bowel sounds using a stethoscope, and assessing additional symptoms such as skin condition and joint pain. These physical examinations give useful information that aids in the diagnosis of Crohn's Disease.

## Diagnostic Tests: Blood Tests, Imaging, Endoscopy

### Blood tests

Blood tests are often used to diagnose Crohn's disease. These tests measure a variety of parameters, including inflammation, dietary deficits, and general organ functioning. Some particular blood tests that may be ordered are:

- **Complete Blood Count (CBC):** This test counts the amount of red, white, and platelet cells in your blood. Anemia (low red blood cell count) and an increased white blood cell count are both typical signs of Crohn's disease inflammation or infection.

- CRP and ESR tests evaluate inflammatory levels in the body. Elevated CRP and ESR values may indicate ongoing inflammation, which is typical of Crohn's Disease.

- Liver function tests assess the health of the liver, which might be impacted by Crohn's disease inflammation or drug side effects.

Imaging studies

Imaging tests help to diagnose Crohn's disease by giving comprehensive pictures of the gastrointestinal system. Common imaging modalities utilized are:

- Ultrasound is a non-invasive imaging technology that employs sound waves to capture pictures of abdominal organs. It may assist detect intestinal irritation, abscesses, and fistulas.

- Computed Tomography (CT) scans provide comprehensive cross-sectional views of the abdomen and pelvis. It detects Crohn's disease-related inflammation, strictures, fistulas, and abscesses.

- Magnetic Resonance Imaging (MRI) provides comprehensive pictures of the gastrointestinal system via the use of magnetic fields and radio waves. They are especially beneficial for examining the small intestine, which is typically affected by Crohn's disease.

## Endoscopy

Endoscopic procedures entail inserting a flexible tube with a camera into the gastrointestinal tract to see the digestive system's lining. Common endoscopic techniques used in detecting Crohn's disease are:

- Colonoscopy provides direct sight of the colon and terminal ileum (end of small intestine). During a colonoscopy, tissue samples (biopsies) may be collected for subsequent examination.

- **Upper endoscopy (EGD):** Examines the esophagus, stomach, and duodenum (initial section of small intestine). It may identify Crohn's Disease-related inflammation, ulceration, and other abnormalities.

These diagnostic procedures, together with a comprehensive medical history review and physical examination, are critical for effectively identifying

Crohn's disease. Healthcare practitioners may create an effective treatment plan for each person by integrating clinical evaluations and objective test findings.

# CHAPTER 3

## Treatment Options

## Medications: Anti-Inflammatory, Immune Suppressors, Biologics

### Medications

Crohn's disease is a chronic ailment that needs meticulous treatment to keep symptoms under control and avoid flare-ups. Medications are essential in treating this illness, to reduce inflammation in the digestive system and alleviate symptoms including stomach discomfort, diarrhea, and exhaustion.

Anti-inflammatory medications are a key component of Crohn's disease therapy. These drugs operate by lowering inflammation in the intestines, which helps to relieve symptoms and avoid consequences. Aminosalicylates (such as mesalamine) and corticosteroids (such as prednisone) are two common anti-inflammatory medications. These drugs may be administered orally, topically, or intravenously, depending on the severity of the symptoms and the level of inflammation.

Immune Suppressors: Another kind of drug used to treat Crohn's disease is an immune suppressant. These medications act by inhibiting the immune system, which may help decrease inflammation and protect the gut lining. Immune suppressors are often recommended to individuals who do not react well to anti-inflammatory drugs or have repeated flare-ups. Immune suppressors include azathioprine, methotrexate, and cyclosporine.

Biologic treatments are a novel kind of drug that has transformed the treatment of Crohn's disease. These medications are generated from live creatures and act by targeting certain immune system proteins that cause inflammation. Biologics are normally reserved for individuals with moderate to severe Crohn's disease who have not responded to previous therapies. Biologic medications used to treat Crohn's disease include infliximab, adalimumab, and ustekinumab.

## Lifestyle Changes: Diet, Exercise, Stress Management

**Lifestyle Changes**

In addition to drugs, lifestyle adjustments may help manage Crohn's disease and improve quality of life. These adjustments might include dietary changes, exercise routines, and stress management approaches.

Diet: Diet may have a substantial influence on Crohn's disease symptoms, however exact dietary advice may differ from person to person. In general, people with Crohn's disease should consume a well-balanced diet rich in fruits and vegetables, healthy grains, and lean meats. Some Crohn's disease patients may have symptoms when they consume dairy products, high-fiber diets, or spicy foods. Keeping a food diary may assist in identifying trigger foods and allow for diet modifications as needed.

**Exercise:** Regular exercise is beneficial to general health and may help control Crohn's symptoms. Exercise may assist in relieving stress, boosting mood, and supporting proper digestion. Walking, swimming, and yoga are all low-impact workouts that will not increase symptoms. However, before beginning any new fitness plan, you should contact with a healthcare practitioner, particularly if you have active Crohn's disease symptoms.

**Stress Management:** Because stress may worsen Crohn's disease symptoms, it's important to learn efficient stress management practices. This might involve deep breathing exercises, meditation, or mindfulness activities. Furthermore, identifying appropriate stress relief activities, such as hobbies or spending time with loved ones, may assist enhance general well-being and lessen the influence of stress on Crohn's symptoms.

## Surgery: When And Why

### Surgery

While drugs and lifestyle adjustments may typically help control Crohn's disease, some individuals may need surgery to alleviate problems or enhance their quality of life.

Surgery for Crohn's disease may be required in a variety of scenarios, including severe inflammation that does not respond to treatments, intestinal blockages, fistulas (abnormal connections between organs), and abscesses (collections of pus). Surgery may also be advised if drugs are no longer helpful or if there is a danger of major consequences such as intestinal perforation or malignancy.

**Forms of Surgery:** Depending on the individual symptoms and problems, numerous forms of surgery are widely used to treat Crohn's Disease. These may include bowel resection, which removes the diseased segment of the intestine and reconnects the healthy ends, and strictureplasty, which widens restricted portions of the gut without removing tissue. In rare situations, surgery may include the development of a temporary or permanent ostomy, which involves bringing a piece of the intestine to the surface of the abdomen to allow for stool transit or fluid drainage.

**Risks and Considerations:** While surgery may be a successful therapy for Crohn's disease, it does come with risks such as infection, bleeding, and anesthetic issues. Furthermore, surgery may not cure Crohn's disease, and symptoms or new problems may arise over time. Before deciding on surgery, consult with a healthcare practitioner about the possible risks and advantages, as well as thoroughly assess all treatment choices.

In conclusion, Crohn's disease therapy consists of a mix of drugs, lifestyle adjustments, and, in some circumstances, surgery. Crohn's disease patients may successfully control their symptoms and enhance their quality of life by working closely with healthcare specialists and adhering to a complete treatment plan.

# CHAPTER 4

## Managing Symptoms

### Dealing With Flare-Ups

Dealing with flare-ups is an important part of managing Crohn's disease. These episodes might be unexpected and disruptive, but with the correct strategy, you can reduce their influence on your regular life. When you're experiencing a flare-up, it's critical to connect with your healthcare team right away. They may provide advice targeted to your unique condition, such as changes to your drug regimen or extra therapies to help manage the flare-up.

Common symptoms during a flare-up include stomach discomfort, diarrhea, exhaustion, and lack of appetite. It's important to listen to your body and rest as required.

Avoiding triggers, such as particular meals or stressful circumstances, may also help reduce symptoms. Additionally, keeping hydrated is critical during flare-ups, since diarrhea may cause dehydration. Drinking enough fluids, such as water, herbal teas, and electrolyte-rich beverages, may aid in replenishing lost fluids and electrolytes.

In extreme circumstances, hospitalization may be required to adequately manage a flare-up. If difficulties emerge, this may include intravenous fluids, nutritional assistance, and, in certain cases, surgery. It is critical to follow your healthcare provider's advice and maintain in connection with them throughout the flare-up and recovery phase.

## Coping With Pain And Discomfort

Pain and discomfort are frequent Crohn's Disease symptoms, however, there are some helpful coping tactics.

Medications provided by your doctor, such as anti-inflammatory medications or pain relievers, may help decrease discomfort and inflammation in the digestive system. It is critical that you take these drugs as prescribed and speak with your healthcare provider if you have any adverse effects or concerns.

In addition to medicine, various strategies may be used to alleviate pain and suffering. Deep breathing, meditation, and yoga are all relaxation exercises that may help decrease stress and tension, which can worsen symptoms. Heat treatment, such as heating pads or warm baths, may also help to relieve stomach discomfort and cramps.

A healthy lifestyle may also help to manage the pain and suffering associated with Crohn's disease. Regular exercise may assist in enhancing general physical and mental health, decreasing inflammation, and relieving stress. Eating a well-balanced diet high in nutrients and low in trigger foods may also help to improve digestive health and alleviate symptoms.

## Nutritional Support

Nutritional assistance is essential for treating Crohn's disease since it may help relieve symptoms, improve healing, and avoid malnutrition. During flare-ups, it is critical to concentrate on meals that are readily digested and mild on the digestive system. This might include bland meals like rice, bananas, applesauce, boiled potatoes, and lean meats like chicken or fish.

In rare circumstances, nutritional supplements or meal replacement shakes may be prescribed to guarantee appropriate nutrient intake during flare-ups or times of low appetite.

These supplements may give necessary vitamins, minerals, and calories to aid in healing and avoid nutritional deficits.

Working with a registered dietitian who specializes in gastrointestinal diseases may help you build a customized nutrition plan based on your specific requirements and preferences. They may help you discover trigger foods, organize your meals, and manage particular symptoms like diarrhea or stomach discomfort.

In addition to dietary modifications, staying hydrated means drinking enough fluids throughout the day. Water is the greatest option, but herbal teas, coconut water, and electrolyte-rich sports drinks may also help you stay hydrated.

By adopting these tactics into your daily routine, you may successfully control Crohn's disease symptoms while also improving your overall quality of life. Working closely with your healthcare team and taking a proactive approach to self-care may help you overcome the difficulties of living with this chronic disease.

# CHAPTER 5

## Diet And Nutrition

## Foods To Avoid

Understanding which foods to avoid while treating Crohn's disease is critical for symptom management and general wellness. While triggers differ from person to person, some foods are known to worsen symptoms and should be avoided. High-fiber meals, such as fresh fruits and vegetables, whole grains, nuts, and seeds, might be especially difficult for Crohn's patients since they can exacerbate diarrhea, stomach discomfort, and bloating. These meals are tough to digest and might aggravate the already irritated intestinal lining.

Furthermore, dairy items such as milk, cheese, and ice cream may cause symptoms in certain people. Lactose intolerance is frequent in people with Crohn's disease, causing gas, bloating, and diarrhea after eating dairy. Fried and fatty meals should also be avoided since they might aggravate diarrhea and cause pain.

Spicy meals and coffee are two more causes that may exacerbate symptoms for certain individuals. Spices may irritate the digestive system, causing further irritation and pain. Caffeine, present in coffee, tea, and certain sodas, may increase bowel movements and aggravate diarrhea in sensitive people.

Alcohol is another thing to avoid or moderate, since it may irritate the gut lining and cause flare-ups in certain people. Carbonated drinks may also cause gas and bloating, which may exacerbate pain.

People with Crohn's disease must pay attention to their bodies' reactions to various meals and discover particular triggers. While the items listed above are often related to aggravating symptoms, the particular triggers vary greatly across people. Keeping a food diary and consulting with a healthcare physician or nutritionist may help you identify problematic items and create a specific diet plan.

## Foods To Include

Building a diet that promotes digestive health and reduces symptoms is critical for successful Crohn's disease management. While trigger foods should be avoided, several nutritional alternatives may help reduce symptoms and enhance general well-being. A Crohn's-friendly diet should contain the following foods:

To begin, eating meals that are easy to digest and low in fiber may help lessen the likelihood of symptoms worsening. Cooked fruits and vegetables, such as peeled and cooked carrots, squash, and applesauce, are easier on the digestive system than raw ones. Similarly, refined carbohydrates such as white rice, white bread, and pasta may deliver energy while remaining comfortable.

A Crohn's-friendly diet includes lean proteins such as skinless chicken, fish, eggs, and tofu. These meals provide vital elements such as protein, iron, and B vitamins, which are necessary for general health and recovery. Incorporating healthy fats such as avocado, and olive oil, and fatty seafood like salmon may also help with nutrient absorption and inflammation.

Probiotic-rich foods, such as yogurt, kefir, and fermented vegetables like sauerkraut and kimchi, may help maintain a healthy gut flora balance. Probiotics may decrease inflammation and improve digestive function in certain Crohn's disease patients.

Furthermore, keeping hydrated is essential for treating symptoms and maintaining overall health. Drinking enough water throughout the day may help avoid dehydration, which occurs often during Crohn's disease flare-ups. Herbal teas and homemade broths may also give soothing hydration without aggravating symptoms.

Finally, including modest, frequent meals in your daily routine might assist avoid overloading the digestive system and alleviating pain. Eating smaller meals more regularly may also assist in guaranteeing appropriate nutritional intake, especially during times of low appetite or flare-ups.

Individuals with Crohn's disease may build a balanced and supportive diet by concentrating on nutrient-dense, readily digested foods and paying attention to specific triggers. This diet helps control symptoms and supports overall health.

## Meal Planning Tips

Meal planning may be a useful tool for people with Crohn's disease since it helps them negotiate dietary issues and ensure they obtain the nutrients they need while reducing discomfort. Here are some useful meal-planning suggestions for treating Crohn's disease:

1. **Maintain a Food Diary:** Tracking food consumption and symptoms may aid in identifying trigger foods and trends. Take note of everything you consume, how much you eat, and any symptoms you encounter afterward. This may assist in identifying problematic items and suggest dietary changes.

2. **Focus on Variety:** Include a variety of meals from various dietary categories to ensure you obtain a diverse range of nutrients.

Experiment with various fruits, veggies, meats, and grains to make meals more exciting and nutrition-dense.

3. Preparing meals and snacks ahead of time will make healthy eating more convenient. Wash and slice fruits and vegetables, prepare grains and meats, and plan snacks for the week.

4. **Consider Texture:** Pay attention to food texture and how it affects digestion. During flare-ups, choose softer, more digestible meals such as smoothies, soups, and well-cooked grains. As symptoms ease, gradually return to harder textures.

5. **Remind Hydrated:** Drink lots of water throughout the day to remain hydrated and help your digestion. Herbal teas, homemade broths, and fruits and vegetables high in water may all help you stay hydrated.

**6. Plan for Snacks:** Keep nutrient-dense snacks on hand in case you are hungry in between meals. Healthy snacks include nuts and seeds, yogurt, fruit, rice cakes with nut butter, and homemade trail mix.

**7. Listen to Your Body:** Pay attention to hunger and fullness signals and eat to meet your body's demands. Be cautious of food amounts and prevent overeating, which may strain the digestive system.

**8. Consult a Dietitian:** Work with a registered dietitian who specializes in gastrointestinal health to create a tailored food plan that fits your nutritional requirements while also addressing your triggers and symptoms.

Individuals with Crohn's disease may use these meal planning suggestions to better negotiate dietary issues, manage symptoms, and improve overall health and well-being.

## CHAPTER 6

## Living With Crohn's Disease

## Maintaining Quality Of Life

Living with Crohn's Disease brings unique obstacles, yet aggressive treatment allows you to retain a good quality of life. One critical component is sticking to your treatment plan. This usually entails using drugs to control symptoms and avoid flare-ups. Your healthcare practitioner will adjust your therapy depending on the severity of your problem, so talk honestly about your symptoms and any changes you see.

In addition to medicine, maintaining a healthy lifestyle may have a big impact. This involves eating a balanced diet that is easy on your digestive system. While trigger foods differ from person to person, many people find comfort in avoiding hot, fatty, or high-fiber meals during flare-ups. Staying hydrated is also important, since dehydration may exacerbate symptoms. Regular exercise may help relieve stress and improve general well-being, but you must choose activities that do not worsen your symptoms.

Managing stress is another important aspect of sustaining quality of life with Crohn's disease. Stress may cause flare-ups and increase symptoms, so developing appropriate coping strategies is critical. Mindfulness meditation, deep breathing exercises, and yoga are all effective stress-reduction techniques. Furthermore, having a support network of understanding friends, family, and healthcare professionals may give emotional support during difficult times.

Regular monitoring of your condition is vital for avoiding any flare-ups. Keep note of your symptoms, triggers, and any changes in your condition, and convey them to your healthcare physician. They may modify your treatment plan as necessary to keep your symptoms under control and avoid consequences.

## Support Networks And Resources

Navigating life with Crohn's Disease may be difficult at times, but you don't have to do it alone. Creating a support network of understanding people may give important emotional and practical help. This network may include friends, family members, support groups, and Crohn's disease-specific internet communities.

Support groups provide a secure environment in which to share experiences, learn from others, and get encouragement. Hearing from others who understand what you're going through may be soothing and reassuring. Online forums and social media groups may also be useful sources of knowledge and support, enabling you to connect with Crohn's Disease patients all over the globe.

In addition to peer support, there are several services available to assist you cope with Crohn's disease. Educational resources, books, and websites include useful information on symptoms, treatments, and coping methods. Your healthcare professional may also give advice and direct you to further resources as required.

When faced with obstacles linked to your disease, do not hesitate to seek assistance. Whether you want aid with everyday duties, emotional support, or practical guidance, there are people and services available to help you along your Crohn's Disease journey.

## Mental Health And Well-Being

Living with a chronic disease, such as Crohn's Disease, may hurt your mental health, but there are actions you can do to improve your situation. It's critical to recognize and handle the emotional consequences of your disease. Individuals with Crohn's Disease often suffer frustration, worry, and sadness, but these emotions do not have to define their experience.

Seeking help from a mental health expert may be quite useful. Therapy may offer a safe area for you to explore your emotions, acquire coping methods, and build resilience in the face of setbacks. Cognitive-behavioral therapy (CBT) is very helpful in reducing stress and anxiety caused by chronic disease.

In addition to professional help, self-care techniques are essential for preserving mental health. Prioritize things that offer you pleasure and relaxation, such as spending time with loved ones, pursuing hobbies, or practicing mindfulness. Taking care of your physical health, such as getting adequate sleep and exercising, helps you feel better overall.

Educating yourself about your disease may help reduce worry and give you the ability to take charge of your health. Understanding your treatment choices, possible consequences, and symptom-management tactics may help you feel more in control.

Finally, don't underestimate the value of connections. Surround yourself with supportive friends, family, and healthcare professionals who will affirm and encourage you. Remember that you are not alone in your battle with Crohn's Disease, and asking for assistance is a show of strength, not weakness. Prioritizing your mental health and well-being allows you to create resilience and flourish in the face of adversities.

# CHAPTER 7

## Complications Of Crohn's Disease

### Fistulas, Abscesses, And Strictures

Fistulas, abscesses, and strictures are some of the most difficult consequences that people with Crohn's disease may encounter. Let's go at each of these concerns to better understand their consequences and management.

Fistulas are abnormal passageways that occur between two or more organs or between an organ and skin. Fistulas are common in Crohn's Disease due to digestive tract inflammation. They may appear anywhere, from the intestines to the skin around the anus. Fistulas may produce symptoms such as discomfort, drainage, and infection. Fistulas are often managed with a mix of anti-inflammatory medicine, antibiotics to prevent infection, and, in rare cases, surgical intervention to repair or seal the fistula.

Abscesses are pus-filled pockets that occur inside the body due to infection. Abscesses may form in the abdominal cavity or around the anus in Crohn's disease. They often produce symptoms including extreme pain, fever, and edema. The abscess is normally treated by draining it via a minimally invasive method or surgery. Antibiotics are also administered to treat the illness and prevent recurrence.

Strictures are narrowings or constrictions in the digestive system that may block the passage of food and feces. Strictures in Crohn's Disease are often caused by prolonged intestinal inflammation and scarring. Symptoms of strictures include stomach discomfort, bloating, and trouble passing stools. Medication to decrease inflammation and dilation operations to enlarge the intestine's constricted segments may be used in treatment. In rare situations, surgery may be required to remove the strictures and restore normal intestinal function.

## Malnutrition And Vitamin Deficiencies

Malnutrition and vitamin deficiencies are major problems for people with Crohn's disease owing to factors such as poor nutritional absorption and dietary limitations. Addressing these dietary problems is critical for general health and successful illness management.

Malnutrition occurs when the body does not obtain enough nutrients to operate correctly. Malnutrition in Crohn's condition may be caused by malabsorption, a reduction in appetite owing to symptoms such as pain and nausea, and dietary limitations enforced to control the condition. Protein, vitamins, and minerals are common dietary deficits associated with Crohn's disease.

Malnutrition management entails collaborating with a healthcare team, including a dietitian, to create a tailored nutrition plan that meets individual requirements while ensuring optimal nutrient intake via food, supplements, or specialized nutritional formulae.

Vitamin shortages: Vitamin shortages are a major worry for people with Crohn's Disease, owing to decreased absorption in the inflamed intestinal mucosa. Vitamin D, vitamin B12, and folate are all often deficient in people with Crohn's disease. These deficits may cause a variety of symptoms, such as weariness, weakness, and neurological issues. Vitamin supplements and monthly blood tests to evaluate vitamin levels are usual management strategies. In certain circumstances, vitamin injections may be required to guarantee proper absorption.

## Osteoporosis And Bone Health

Osteoporosis, a disorder marked by weaker and brittle bones, is a possible consequence of Crohn's Disease, owing to variables such as inflammation, malnutrition, and the use of corticosteroid medicines. Maintaining bone health is critical for Crohn's patients to avoid fractures and other consequences.

Bone Density Monitoring: Crohn's disease patients should have frequent bone density tests to determine their risk of osteoporosis. These procedures, such as dual-energy X-ray absorptiometry (DEXA) scans, assess bone density and detect indicators of bone loss or osteoporosis. Based on the findings, healthcare experts may make appropriate recommendations to avoid additional bone degradation.

Adopting lifestyle changes to enhance bone health is critical for people with Crohn's disease. This includes doing weight-bearing activities like walking or strength training, which assist in strengthening bones and lower the risk of fracture. Additionally, maintaining bone density requires enough calcium and vitamin D consumption via food and supplements.

Medication Management: In certain situations, healthcare experts may recommend drugs to prevent or treat osteoporosis in Crohn's disease patients. These drugs, such as bisphosphonates and selective estrogen receptor modulators (SERMs), serve to enhance bone density and lower the risk of fracture. However, the usage of these drugs should be carefully supervised, taking into account individual risk factors and possible adverse effects.

Individuals with Crohn's Disease may significantly reduce the impact of these issues on their overall health and quality of life by treating them and applying suitable treatment techniques. Regular monitoring, communication with healthcare experts, and commitment to treatment programs are critical components of addressing these complicated conditions.

# CHAPTER 8

## Pregnancy And Crohn's Disease

### Fertility Issues

Understanding the relationship between Crohn's disease and fertility is critical for anybody wanting a family. While Crohn's disease does not directly influence fertility, several variables linked with the illness might make conception more difficult. Pelvic inflammation, surgical scarring, and Crohn's disease drugs may all influence fertility.

Those with Crohn's disease who are attempting to conceive must discuss freely with both their gastroenterologist and obstetrician. Your gastroenterologist can explain how your Crohn's disease is presently controlled and any possible concerns linked with pregnancy.

They may also propose changes to your treatment plan to ensure it is safe during pregnancy.

## Pregnancy Management

Managing Crohn's disease during pregnancy needs close collaboration between you, your gastroenterologist, and your obstetrician. One of the most important concerns is medicine. Some drugs used to treat Crohn's disease may be unsafe during pregnancy, while others are deemed low risk. Your gastroenterologist can assist you in deciding which drugs to take, which to alter, and which to discontinue completely during pregnancy.

Regular monitoring is another important part of controlling Crohn's disease during pregnancy. Your healthcare team will most likely plan more regular check-ups to evaluate both your Crohn's symptoms and the health of the baby. These check-ups may involve blood testing, stool tests, and imaging tests such as ultrasounds to monitor your health and guarantee your baby's appropriate development.

Dietary issues are extremely crucial during pregnancy, particularly for those who have Crohn's disease. While there is no one-size-fits-all diet for Crohn's disease, being aware of what you eat and how it affects your symptoms may help you remain healthy throughout pregnancy. To assist manage your Crohn's symptoms while pregnant, see your gastroenterologist or certified dietitian about which foods to eat and which to avoid.

## Risks And Precautions

Pregnancy for women with Crohn's Disease, like any other, has certain hazards. One cause for worry is illness flares, which may develop during pregnancy owing to hormonal and immune system changes. Flares may cause issues for both the mother and the baby, so it's important to coordinate with your healthcare team to monitor your status and change your treatment plan as required.

Another danger is a higher possibility of premature delivery and low birth weight. Women with active Crohn's Disease are more likely to have these issues, thus it is critical to adequately treat your illness during pregnancy to limit the risk. This may include prescription modifications, dietary changes, and regular monitoring by your healthcare team.

Furthermore, some women with Crohn's illness may need surgery during pregnancy if they develop problems such as intestinal blockages or severe illness flares. While surgery during pregnancy is uncommon and should be avoided whenever feasible, it may be essential in certain cases to safeguard the health of both the mother and the baby.

# CHAPTER 9

## Children And Crohn's Disease

## Pediatric Considerations

Crohn's disease may affect people of all ages, including youngsters. Understanding how the illness develops in pediatric patients is critical to optimal care. Crohn's disease symptoms in children can include stomach discomfort, diarrhea, weight loss, and exhaustion. Diagnosing Crohn's disease in children, on the other hand, might be difficult since the symptoms coincide with those of other prevalent juvenile disorders.

One of the most important aspects of pediatric Crohn's disease is its influence on growth and development. Children with Crohn's disease may face development delays as a result of poor nutrition absorption, persistent inflammation, and adverse effects from illness-management drugs.

Healthcare practitioners must regularly monitor children's growth and intervene with appropriate therapies to promote normal development.

## Growth And Development

Children with Crohn's disease may experience specific developmental obstacles. Chronic inflammation in the digestive system might reduce nutritional absorption, resulting in growth deficits. Furthermore, using corticosteroids and other drugs to treat Crohn's disease may hurt bone health and height potential.

To address these issues, healthcare experts may propose dietary treatments to ensure that children with Crohn's disease get enough calories, protein, vitamins, and minerals for healthy development. This may include dietary changes, such as boosting calorie and protein consumption, as well as supplementation with vitamins and minerals that are deficient owing to malabsorption.

Regular monitoring of growth metrics, including height, weight, and body mass index (BMI), is critical for detecting development delays early and implementing effective treatments. In rare situations, children with severe growth limitations may need specialist treatment from a pediatric gastroenterologist or a multidisciplinary team to manage their complicated dietary requirements and maximize development potential.

## Treatment Approaches

Treating Crohn's disease in children requires a specialized strategy that considers their specific needs and problems. The therapy aims to induce and sustain remission, ease symptoms, promote normal growth and development, and reduce the risk of complications.

Medications are often the foundation of therapy for pediatric Crohn's disease. Anti-inflammatory treatments like mesalamine, immunomodulators like azathioprine and methotrexate, and biologic therapy like infliximab and adalimumab are all widely utilized. The choice of medicine is determined by criteria such as illness severity, response to prior therapies, and the occurrence of problems.

In addition to drugs, dietary treatment may be effective in controlling Crohn's disease in children. Exclusive enteral nutrition (EEN), which consists of drinking a liquid formula as the only source of nourishment for an extended period, has been demonstrated to elicit remission and increase growth in juvenile Crohn's patients. Nutritional treatment may be used alone or in conjunction with drugs to produce the best results.

Surgery may be required for children with severe Crohn's disease complications such as strictures, fistulas, or abscesses that do not respond to medication treatment. Surgical procedures are intended to remove damaged parts of the gut, relieve symptoms, and enhance quality of life. However, surgery is usually reserved for situations when medical care has failed or consequences are severe.

Overall, treating Crohn's disease in children requires a multidisciplinary approach combining pediatric gastroenterologists, dietitians, surgeons, and other healthcare providers. Addressing the special requirements of juvenile Crohn's patients and customizing treatment options to their circumstances will enhance the results and quality of life for these young patients.

# CHAPTER 10

## Research And Future Perspectives

## Advances In Crohn's Disease Research

Crohn's disease research has advanced significantly in recent years, bringing promise for better knowledge, therapy, and, eventually, management of the disorder. Scientists and medical experts throughout the globe are working to understand the complexity of Crohn's disease to create more effective medications and ultimately discover a cure.

Genetics is one area of concentration in research. Researchers are investigating the genetic variables that contribute to the development of Crohn's disease, to identify particular genes connected with the disorder. Understanding the genetic foundation of Crohn's disease may lead to more individualized treatment options that are matched to each individual's genetic makeup.

Another important part of Crohn's disease research is the study of the gut flora. The gut microbiota is vital for gut health and immune system regulation. Researchers are looking at how changes in the gut microbiota may influence the development and course of Crohn's disease. This study opens the door to potential therapy techniques that target the gut microbiota to successfully control Crohn's disease.

Furthermore, advances in imaging technology have transformed the diagnosis and surveillance of Crohn's Disease. High-resolution imaging methods like magnetic resonance imaging (MRI) and capsule endoscopy give precise views of the gastrointestinal system, allowing healthcare providers to more correctly monitor disease activity and consequences.

Furthermore, research into the immunological systems that underpin Crohn's disease continues to provide vital insights. Understanding how immune system dysregulation leads to intestinal inflammation in Crohn's disease allows researchers to design tailored immunomodulatory medicines that restore immunological balance and reduce disease symptoms.

## Promising Therapies On The Horizon

Exciting improvements in Crohn's disease therapy are on the horizon, giving patients hope for better results and a higher quality of life. Several intriguing medicines are now being studied, with the potential to change Crohn's disease treatment.

Biological medicines, such as monoclonal antibodies that target particular molecules involved in the inflammatory process, have altered the therapy options for Crohn's disease.

Ongoing research seeks to create next-generation biologics with improved effectiveness and safety profiles, providing patients with additional alternatives for individualized therapy.

Furthermore, small molecule inhibitors of critical inflammatory pathways are being developed as an alternate therapy for Crohn's disease. These oral drugs provide more convenience and flexibility than conventional biologics, possibly enhancing treatment adherence and patient outcomes.

Stem cell treatment is another novel technique for treating Crohn's disease. Researchers hope to heal damaged intestinal tissue and restore normal gut function in Crohn's disease patients by tapping into stem cells' regenerative potential. Early clinical studies have shown encouraging results, indicating that stem cell therapy might revolutionize the treatment of Crohn's disease in the future.

Furthermore, tailored medicine techniques are gaining popularity in Crohn's disease therapy. Healthcare practitioners may adapt treatment strategies to improve results while minimizing adverse effects by taking into account individual patient characteristics such as genetic predisposition, illness phenotype, and response to medication.

## Advocacy And Awareness Efforts

Advocacy and awareness activities are critical in increasing knowledge of Crohn's disease, campaigning for better patient treatment and support, and moving research forward. Various organizations, patient advocacy groups, and healthcare professionals are actively engaged in advocacy efforts to ensure that the needs of people living with Crohn's disease are met efficiently.

These advocacy activities are focused on many critical areas, including raising public awareness of Crohn's disease and its effects on people and families. Advocacy groups want to minimize stigma and misunderstanding regarding Crohn's disease by promoting knowledge of its symptoms, diagnosis, and treatment choices.

Furthermore, advocacy organizations work persistently to support legislation and initiatives that promote affordable healthcare and treatment alternatives for Crohn's disease patients. This involves fighting for insurance coverage for necessary drugs and treatments, as well as increasing research funding to increase scientific knowledge and treatment development.

Furthermore, advocacy activities attempt to enable people with Crohn's disease to take an active role in their healthcare. Advocacy groups assist people with Crohn's disease by offering resources, support networks, and educational materials to help them negotiate the obstacles of managing their illness and make educated healthcare choices.

To summarize, advocacy and awareness initiatives are critical for advancing Crohn's disease research, treatment, and support. We can make a significant impact in the lives of millions throughout the globe by working together to promote awareness, lobby for better treatment, and empower Crohn's disease patients.

# CONCLUSION

In conclusion, Crohn's Disease is a complicated and chronic ailment that has a tremendous influence on individuals who suffer from it. Throughout this investigation, it has become clear that the specific causation of Crohn's Disease is unknown, with a mix of genetic, environmental, and immunological variables contributing to its development. The disease's heterogeneity complicates diagnosis and therapy, necessitating a multidisciplinary approach combining gastroenterologists, dietitians, surgeons, and other healthcare specialists.

Despite advances in medical knowledge and therapy alternatives, controlling Crohn's disease is a dynamic and continuing process. While immunosuppressants, biologics, and corticosteroids may help reduce inflammation and ease symptoms, they are not without dangers and adverse effects.

Surgical procedures may be required in the event of problems or when drugs are inadequate.

Furthermore, the effects of Crohn's Disease go beyond physical symptoms, impacting mental well-being, social relationships, and general quality of life. Coping with a chronic disease requires perseverance, social support, and access to mental health services.

Crohn's Disease research continues to provide new insights into its pathophysiology, biomarkers for early identification, and innovative treatment techniques. As the medical world works toward tailored and targeted methods, such as precision medicine and microbiome-based therapeutics, there is promise for better results and a higher quality of life for Crohn's patients.

Finally, promoting awareness, pushing for increased access to healthcare services, and creating a friendly atmosphere for Crohn's Disease patients are critical steps toward resolving the condition's problems. We may strive toward a better understanding, treatment, and, eventually, a cure for Crohn's Disease by cooperating across disciplines and providing people with information and tools.

**THE END**

www.ingramcontent.com/pod-product-compliance
Lightning Source LLC
Chambersburg PA
CBHW070317230526
45470CB00002B/917